TIME TO HYDRATE !

A new water-based health method

SIBYL BALADI, Ph.D.

i

DEDICATION

In loving memory of my mother.
I am forever grateful for her unwavering support
and encouragement in the creation of this book.

Table of Contents

1 Introduction

I suffered from a health problem for several years when I shouldn't have. And I am certainly not the only one in this situation.

Indeed, we all suffer some day during our life from one or from several avoidable diseases. For some people, it will just be a cold, for others it will be a rash or hypertension, or in the worst case, cancer. For me, it was gastrointestinal problems. Several years ago, I started to suffer from digestive issues almost every day although as a child or as a teenager I didn't have such problems. I thus resolved to eat lots of rice, since rice constipates. And since things did not get any better, I decided to see my doctor. I remember that, during my first visit, the doctor asked me to describe my diet, such as the schedule of my meals (i.e., whether I regularly ate at breakfast, lunch and dinner), or the quality of my meals (particularly if I quickly swallowed a sandwich due to lack of time during my lunch breaks at work). I replied to him that not only did I eat regularly but that I also took the time to eat.

Although this happened several years ago, I remember his diagnosis very well, which was surprising yet credible: stress. "You know the saying, he said, 'soil your pants'. All this is due to stress and anxiety. Your digestion problems are probably due to this: stress". At the time, I believed him since I was indeed extremely stressed out due to personal problems. I was moreover young and influenceable. Besides, my young age probably incited my doctor not to prescribe tranquilizers, or he did not consider this necessary. He nevertheless recommended a treatment based on dietary fiber supplements, which I followed but without achieving the expected success.

Yet, I am today extremely surprised that he never asked me whether I regularly drank enough water, as I am now persuaded that my digestion issues were simply due to a lack of water in my body. Indeed, I seem to remember that I didn't drink much water, probably because of my rather frequent need to urinate, perhaps due to too small a bladder. Besides, my stress level probably didn't help, since I did not think about hydrating myself sufficiently.

This state of constant under-hydration (or

even dehydration) was most likely the reason for the failure of my recovery despite the dietary fiber treatment, and I am now sure that had my doctor advised me to drink more water, my digestive disorder would have been rapidly cured. Unfortunately, one has to admit that not only physicians but also dentists rarely advise us to drink more water so as to stay in good health. Indeed, I recently noticed that many of my friends and family members, who see doctors for various ailments such as bursitis (inflammation of the fluid-filled pads at the joints), fasciitis plantaris (inflammation of the tissue that supports the arch of the foot), migraines of moderate intensity, or for other diseases of mild conditions not only do not drink enough water, but have not been advised by their doctor to hydrate themselves more. This is actually an important even crucial point, since drinking water is vital.

One may wonder why doctors do not incite us to drink more water to cure diseases, even to prevent them. Is this due to shortcomings of the university system? Medical students probably learn in academia lists of diseases with their respective medicines, but they are maybe not taught to advise their future patients to drink enough water every day. Or, doctors simply do not think of suggesting to their patients to hydrate more, either because it seems trivial, or because they themselves do not drink enough water. Or else, they may even fear that their patients might be opposed to their recommendation, or even complain about it, because this would force them to go more frequently to the toilet, so as to eliminate the excess water consumed based on their advice. Finally, one may wonder whether doctors simply assume that their patients drink the recommended amount of fluids and are not chronically dehydrated.

In any case, during my visits at his office, my doctor never suggested I drink water for my digestive problems and, most importantly, he did not suggest the method that I will present in this book.

This health method is for everyone: men, women, the young and the older, and particularly for the elderly and for people suffering from one or even from several ailments that they wish to cure, or who fear going to the toilet too often during the day or even at night.

2 The water-based health method

I heard from many people, both young (in their thirties) and older (from 70 to 80 years old), but particularly men over 40 and women of all ages: "if I drink I frequently go to the toilet", or "if I drink before going to bed, I have to wake up during the night".

This was actually my case, since several years ago I frequently used the bathroom. I even woke up at night sometimes more than once, to relieve my bladder. I thought that it was simply due to the fact that I was a woman with a small bladder, since women usually have a smaller bladder than men due to the uterus, which takes up space near the bladder. Most women therefore have to empty their bladder more frequently than men. This would actually explain the lines that form in front of the women's restrooms, whereas men rarely line up in front of the restrooms (from what I have been told and what I could see from outside).

The problem is that people's first reaction, so as to avoid going to the bathroom too often, is to avoid drinking too much. This represents a major error that must be corrected at all costs.

During (too) many years, I made this mistake myself by minimizing my intake of water for fear of constantly going to the toilet, particularly in places without restrooms (for example during road trips or at the beach, etc.).

The more I minimized my water intake, the more my body was dehydrated, without my realizing it. One day, I probably stopped drinking enough water to hydrate my body, which may have been in a state of constant dehydration, which probably triggered my digestive problems. This may have probably turned into a vicious circle, the less I drank and the less I digested well, which paradoxically made me urinate frequently. And the more I dreaded going to the bathroom, the less I drank for fear of going to the toilet all the time. The physiological explanation is hard to grasp. My entire body must have been in a state of total imbalance and my large intestine could no longer perform its major function, that is the adequate absorption of water inside my body, which may have prevented it from functioning properly.

Ever since I have applied my new health method with water (presented in detail in the following paragraphs), my body has regained a healthy balance, and I can hydrate myself without being afraid of going to the toilet often (or of having to wake up during the night to empty my bladder), and, above all, by ensuring that my entire body is in optimal shape (including my skin, which, by being continuously hydrated, radiates and looks younger, and also all my internal organs, as well as my teeth, my nails and my hair).

If this method was successful for me, it will most likely prove successful for everyone, including all who read this book.

This new water-based health method simply consists of taking a sip of water at frequent and regular intervals, and this all day long until bedtime. This continuous hydration method by small fractions enables the body to constantly stay hydrated, without provoking the need to urinate often. Indeed, the regular intake of water in small amounts allows water to diffuse slowly and gradually in the body. This irrigates the body optimally and long-lastingly, and thereby all the cells of the organs, and prevents water to pass directly (and rapidly) into the bladder, where it is then eliminated without being able to perform its beneficial and vital role of hydration and cleansing of the organism.

Given that this new water-based health method is built on a continuous hydration of the body thanks to a frequent and regular intake of sips of water, it is recommended to start by taking one sip of water every thirty minutes and then modify, if required, the frequency of the water sip consumption. This thirty minute-duration, which represents the base frequency of the intake of water sips, is the result of an empirical approach: fifteen minutes represents a period of time slightly too short during which the sips of water, being too close together cannot fulfill their function of progressive and optimal hydration of the organism, whereas one hour constitutes a duration that is slightly too long, causing sips of water too far apart in time and not allowing an optimal and constant body hydration.

As to the sips of water, they should be taken naturally and it is not necessary to modify their volume. We just have to take a sip of water and feel the liquid flowing down the throat thereby starting the bodily hydration. In contrast, the frequency of the intake of the sips of water should be adjusted individually in order to optimize the water intake in everyone's body, so as to fully hydrate the organism. Indeed, the volume of the sip of water is specific to each individual and depends of the size of the mouth. Thereby, a person with a small mouth will swallow a little bit of water with every sip, whereas a person with a big mouth will probably take a larger sip of water. Everyone has to find the ideal frequency of the intake of sips of water and of the amount of water for his/her/their body and health. Some people will have to take a sip of water every thirty minutes as prescribed by this water-based health method, others will consume a sip of water every twenty minutes, while others could take a sip every 45 minutes. This will depend on each person's metabolism. There isn't really any rules, except having each day enough sips of water approximately every half hour, in order to maximize the body's hydration, without however turning to excess and to a surplus of useless (even harmful) water in the organism.

If preferred, the volume of the sip of water can be adjusted instead of modifying the frequency of the consumption of the sips of water, but it is perhaps easier to diminish or increase the rhythm of the water consumption rather than trying to change the size of the sips of water. That said, everyone should find his/her/their ideal formula to maintain his/her/their body hydrated at all times.

The volume and the frequency of the sips of water will probably vary for each individual (although maybe only slightly) and will be determined based on the results of healing of the dysfunctions and the diseases of the body, as well as on the general health of the organism, meaning the quality of sleep, the state of fatigue, the predisposition to become sick, etc.

So, if a person suffers for example from digestive issues (similar to or different from those from which I suffered), from an inflammatory disease (such as plantar fasciitis or bursitis), from a rash, from depression (mild or even moderate) or from another illness that he or she wishes to cure, and that no improvement is visible after having followed the water-based health method described in this book, it could mean that the minimum amount of water absorbed every day and required by the body, is not reached yet. Either because the sips of water swallowed each time are too small, or because the time lapse between the sips of water is too long. It is then advisable to modify the dose of water consumed by taking sips of water more frequently (for example every 15 minutes) or by taking larger sips of water.

Once the minimal amount of water required by the body is reached, the organism is in its hydric balance and can optimally perform its function of blood circulation, regulation of blood pressure and body temperature, food digestion, elimination of toxins and waste, joint lubrication and of diverse metabolic processes, without producing any stress or inflammation in body tissues or organs. The frequent and regular intake of small amounts of water in the body, thanks to this new health method, keeps the organism in an ideal hydration status. The maintenance of the body hydration is fundamental for both the physical and mental health, and the water-based health method, presented in this book, enables the body to achieve and maintain a water balance, contributing to the preservation of a healthy body in good shape. This new water-based method actually acts as a fountain of youth with purifying and regenerating virtues of water. The water equilibration of the body, thanks to this new hydration method, can however take several weeks or even several months to take effect, or even maybe several years in certain rare cases. One has to be persistent, and it is essential not to give up if the expected healing results are not immediately achieved. The results will often be noticeable over the long term, and one has to be patient and demonstrate perseverance in the accomplishment of this health method and of its frequent and regular intake of sips of water.

In order to maintain the relatively frequent rhythm of the water consumption in small amounts, some people will need to set up a timer or an alarm clock (either manual or an alarm from a cell phone, or even a reminder from a computer's calendar), to remind themselves to take sips of water regularly. Others won't need such a support, because they will easily remember to take a sip of water approximately every half hour by verifying on their watch, or on the clock of their cell phone or their computer. For some, once they will get used to regularly have a sip of water all day long, it will become an automatism and it will no longer be necessary for them to time each consumption of water. They will drink at more or less constant intervals, for example approximately every twenty minutes, or after a time lapse of 15 minutes and then after 30 minutes, without really timing their consumptions of water and without worrying to sip water at fixed time intervals. For others however, it may be difficult to think about taking sips of water at frequent intervals even after practicing the water-based health method for weeks or even months, and they will have to always use an alarm, so as to remind themselves to regularly take sips of water.

It should be specified that this new health method not only requires to drink water frequently and regularly, but also requires to have small sips of water and not whole glasses of water. The consumption of whole glasses of water approximately every half hour may indeed unbalance the organism and prevent an ideal hydration of the body by overloading it with water, which can be harmful (drinking several gallons of water within a few hours is notably dangerous for the brain). This may also cause the need to use the toilet all the time, which is absolutely not the purpose of this new health method.

Furthermore, to properly apply this hydration

method, it isn't necessary to wait to be thirsty to drink some water, but it is important to take one sip of water approximately every thirty minutes all day long, even if we don't feel thirsty at all. It is however essential to take just a sip of water and not more than one sip at a time (except, for example, in case of extreme heat or in case of a delay between each consumption of sips of water exceeding one hour or more, as mentioned later). The intake of small amounts of water is indeed crucial for the success of this health method in order to allow an optimal and continuous hydration of the body without causing frequent needs to urinate.

This new water-based method is relatively simple to follow every day by everyone, except of course for those who work and who don't have the possibility (or the permission) to quench their thirst at work. These people will therefore have to take breaks during their working days, so as to be able to consume sips of water at frequent intervals and thus accomplish this health method effectively. It may, however, not always be possible to take breaks at work every 30 minute (for example for professions practiced in certain hospitals or laboratories, in certain factories, in certain transport vehicles, etc.). In this case, it is necessary to hydrate by taking a small (or even a large) sip of water as soon as the opportunity arises (ideally at most every hour). If the interval between the breaks exceeds one to two hours, it is then preferable to take several sips of water as soon as possible (or even a whole glass of water), so as to reconstitute the body's water reserves lost during these few hours and to sufficiently hydrate the organism, so that it can hold out until the next break without dehydrating too much.

If it is paramount, in this new health method, to frequently and regularly drink water all day, there is however no need to force oneself to drink 48-64 fl. oz of water (or 6 to 8 glasses) as we often hear. Indeed, in order to optimize this hydration method, it is preferable not to count exactly the volume of water consumed every day, nor to force oneself to drink a minimum of 48 fl. oz of water. This can indeed turn out to be too constraining and can moreover be too complicated to do particularly in today's world with its rapid and hectic rhythm. We should rather concentrate on the frequency of the consumption of sips of water. Actually, it is not the daily amount of water that prevails in this health method, but the frequency and the regularity of a continuous hydration thanks to small amounts of water consumed. Obviously, the daily intake of sips of water approximately every thirty minutes, combined with the consumption of coffee or tea in the morning and of beverages at lunch and dinner, will most certainly produce a volume of approximately 48 fl. oz of water, i.e., close to the recommended volume of 48-64 fl. oz mentioned above.

Although the daily consumption of at least 48 fl. oz is not required in this new hydration method, it should be pointed out that in order to prove optimal and thus beneficial, this health method (with frequent intake of sips of water) must be coupled with the consumption of one glass of water (or even more) during lunch and dinner, as well as during breakfast if coffee, tea or fruit juice are not consumed in the morning. Some people think that drinking water during meals dilute digestive juices and disrupts digestion. But this is a myth that should not be perpetuated. It is in fact preferable and even essential to drink water while eating particularly if wine or beer is served with meals (since alcohol dehydrates, as indicated below). The amount of water to consume during meals depends however on each individual. Some will digest better by drinking a big glass of water (or even a full bottle of 16.9 fl. oz). Others, on the other hand, will only need a small glass of water to support digestion. Everyone has to find their optimal dose.

It is important to point out that the water consumption during meals should absolutely not replace the intake of sips of water, but should be associated with the regular consumption of small sips of water, which must imperatively be done first thing in the morning when getting out of bed, then all morning and all afternoon, until the evening just before going to bed. This frequent intake of small sips of water must also be done even if we drink coffee or tea in the morning or during the remaining of the day. Indeed, coffee and tea dehydrate due to their diuretic effects. Water from a coffee or a tea is therefore eliminated more rapidly by the body than pure water. It is therefore recommended to take a few sips of water (or even a full glass of water) within an hour after the consumption of coffee or tea, in order to avoid dehydration of the body.

This also (and mostly) applies if wine, beer or

liquor is consumed, since the consumption of alcohol may lead to a significant dehydration of the organism. It is indeed necessary to always rehydrate the body after drinking alcohol, any alcohol, even after just a beer. Indeed, beer (even though it brings a large amount of water based on the volume absorbed) dehydrates. This dehydrating effect is due to the alcohol present in non-negligible quantity: 4 to 10% depending on the type of beer. The consumption of wine or liquor, which contain even more alcohol than beer (between 10 and 45%, or more for certain alcohols, such as absinthe or certain liquors) requires a fairly rapid rehydration by water in order to maintain the water balance of the body. It is therefore preferable not to wait more than half an hour after their consumption, particularly of course, if we drink, for example whiskey (or any other liquor) neat with no ice. In that case, it is strongly recommended to accompany the glass of whiskey (or of liquor) with a glass of water (called a "water chaser" or a "water back"). In contrast, the consumption of a beer or a cocktail (often mixed with fruit or vegetable juices, with soda or diet soda, with cream, etc., therefore providing water) does not require consuming water as quickly. Just as for coffee or tea, we can probably wait about an hour after a beer or a cocktail – but not much more – before taking a sip of water.

This will however depend once again on each person's metabolism. Some will have to rapidly take a sip of water after one glass of beer or after a cocktail, because they will dehydrate faster than others, who won't require an immediate rehydration of their organism. Everyone will therefore have to adapt the water-based health method according to the dehydration rate of their body caused by alcohol and will have to adjust the frequency of the intake of the sips of water after the consumption of alcohol. Since it can be difficult to evaluate the degree of body dehydration (indeed, except for a dry mouth and the color of urine – the darker the urine, the more dehydrated you are – there isn't really a simple way to measure the level of dehydration), the basic principle of the new water-based health method described in this book should simply be followed and water can be sipped approximately thirty minutes after consuming a beer or a cocktail. Or yet, one can slightly modify the water-based health method and, as indicated above, wait about an hour before taking a sip of water (just like after having coffee or tea).

This health method should also be adjusted based on each person's diet. Indeed, certain fruits and vegetables (such as strawberries, watermelons, tomatoes, cucumbers, etc.), as well as certain meals (such as soups, mashed potatoes, yogurts, etc.) contain a high percentage of water, and therefore represent an excellent source of hydration for the organism. People who eat a lot of watery fruits or vegetables will thus need to take sips of water less frequently than those who eat mainly low-moisture food (such as bread, hard cheese, chocolate or biscuits). By contrast, people who don't eat a lot of high-water content food will have to compensate the lack of water intake from food either by taking sips of water more frequently or by drinking more water during lunch or dinner. Besides, it is generally highly recommended to drink water (even just a sip) each time food is consumed. Indeed, as mentioned above, it is preferable to drink water while eating, since this water intake can help the intestines digest absorbed food, particularly of course when food does not contain a lot of water.

In order to ensure optimal effectiveness of this water-based health method, it is not only necessary to adjust the water consumption according to the food ingested, but also to adjust the water intake depending on the physical effort provided during the day. Thereby, someone who exercises (for example jogs every morning) will have to hydrate much more than someone who is sedentary. Indeed, in order to maintain the body's hydric balance during workouts, and to compensate for water losses (generally high) due to sweating and breathing, it is extremely important to increase the water intake in the body by taking small sips of water, before during and after physical activity. We should in fact follow the example of professional tennis players. Indeed, you may notice during tennis matches that tennis players regularly take a little sip of water or of liquid. It most certainly comes from a desire to keep their body perfectly hydrated, so as to perform well throughout the game, which can sometimes last several hours (the conception of my new water-based health method was actually inspired by this tennis player practice). Just like tennis players, people who practice jogging (or any other endurance sport) should also frequently take small sips of water, for example every 10-15 minutes, during their physical activity sessions. Yet, I often (if not too often) see on the streets joggers in athletic outfits, wearing earbuds in their ears to motivate their run, but without the essential: a small bottle of water (particularly if the jogging session lasts a long time). It is indeed highly recommended to consume water (preferably in small sips) during a fairly intensive workout, like for example jogging or running, since this prevents blood thickening and therefore enables good oxygen transport and tendon lubrication.

Moreover, the consumption of water in small sips enables an optimal hydration of the organism and can prevent the occurrence of cramps, which often results from dehydration of the body. In the case of highly intensive or long duration sports activities, it may even be preferable to have sips of isotonic or sports drinks containing minerals, including sodium, in order to compensate the loss of mineral salts eliminated in sweat and prevent too low a concentration of sodium in the blood (which would produce, by osmotic effect, a hyperhydration inside the body's cells, and thus an imbalance of the organism). It is however necessary to be careful not to drink too much during exercise (even isotonic or sports beverages), so as not to be victim of a water intoxication due to an overconsumption of water, which could generate a brain function disorder (as mentioned above).

In fact, athletes are not the only ones who should carry a bottle of water with them during their activities. Indeed, since the health method described in this book requires taking a small sip of water approximately every half hour (even if we move), it is therefore highly recommended to always bring a bottle of water during travels on foot, by bike or by car. The size of the water bottle will depend on the duration of the trip. Thus, a small bottle of 8 fl. oz will be most suitable for a 1- to 2-hour trip. Whereas it will be preferable to carry a larger bottle (of at least 16.9 fl. oz) for a trip of several hours (particularly of course if it is warm outside). It is however not necessary to bring a bottle of water for just a short walk of half an hour (but it is of course not forbidden, particularly if the walk turns out to be longer than expected). During walks, the water bottle can easily be carried in a backpack, or in a shoulder bag or even in a plastic bag. It is obviously necessary to favor plastic bottles (or preferably aluminum/renewable material ones), so as not to take the risk of breaking glass bottles. It is also advisable to properly close bottle caps before placing the bottles in a bag, so as to prevent the bottle from leaking and the water from wetting the bag and its content. For those who prefer to travel light (i.e., without a bag), there are commercial bottle carrier bags with shoulder straps, as well as running/hydration belts designed for running, equipped with one or several bottle holders. The bottle may also simply be held in the hand (particularly for a short trip). In order to keep water fresh longer (given that water in a plastic bottle will slowly warm up), a vacuum flask (or thermos) can be used preferably with a bottle holder to carry the bottle for example on the shoulder with a handle, or to hang it to a backpack. In the case of very long walks (or during the summer when it is hot outside), it is recommended to purchase cold water bottles along the way, as long as shops that sell refrigerated water bottles are located on the road.

Note that sometimes there is no opportunity to get a bottle of water before going out and we may stay more than an hour without being able to drink (for example if stuck in a traffic jam or in a location without any grocery or convenience stores close by). In this case, it is absolutely necessary to compensate the loss of water incurred by the organism during the period exceeding the interval of approximately thirty minutes recommended by this new health method, by drinking straight, as soon as we have the opportunity, several sips of water (or even a full glass of water, if no water has been consumed for several hours) in order to quench thirst and to rehydrate the body.

Obviously when we feel thirsty, we should always quench our thirst. This can occur (even when fully applying this water-based health method) during heat waves or during extensive physical efforts, such as the jogging mentioned above, or when we are forced to spend several hours without water, as indicated above. Likewise, when salty meals are consumed, it is necessary to compensate with water the intake of salt coming from food in order to equilibrate both the blood sodium level and the water distribution in the organism. In fact, we should satisfy our body with water (and thus all the cells of the lungs, the muscles, the stomach, the intestines, the brain, the skin, etc.) just like we satisfy our body with food (preferably of course without any excess). It should however be noted that if thirst is quenched by drinking in one gulp a large volume of water, soda or any other refreshing beverage, it is then no longer necessary to take a sip of water thirty minutes later. In these conditions, we can probably wait at least one hour before starting to apply again the new water-based health method with its regular and frequent consumption of sips of water. Actually, the water consumption must be in adequacy with the water losses, so as to maintain a bodily hydric balance and prevent a dehydration of the organism.

Finally, it should be pointed out that this new health method, which consists of taking a sip of water approximately every thirty minutes, must of course be followed while we are awake (during the day or the evening) and not while we sleep at night (so as not to affect sleep). It would indeed be unreasonable, or even harmful, not to sleep for the sole purpose of applying this health method. Sometimes, we may however wake up at night unintentionally. It is then preferable, if possible without disrupting sleep too much, to take a small sip of water (or more if we are thirsty or heavily perspiring), so as to replace the losses of water that the body undergoes during these long hours of sleep without hydration. It is however not absolutely necessary to drink water during nighttime awakenings, since the body's metabolism slows down during sleep, and the need for water therefore decreases compared to the need for water while awake, particularly of course if the body has been well hydrated during the day thanks to the water-based health method described in this book.

This new water-based health method can, if optimally applied, contribute to improving physical and mental health, as well as well-being. This new health method may also help cure illnesses or minor diseases, and maybe also malignant diseases (while being treated by a primary or specialty care physician). It is actually recommended to always seek the advice of a medical professional in case of a serious illness (or relatively serious, or even in case of a benign disease). A general practitioner or physician specialist can indeed provide medical advice on a case-by-case basis, so as to help improve everyone's health and wellness while drinking water as described in this chapter.

3 The diseases generated by the lack of water

Water is not only a main constituent of the human body (which is made of some 60 to 70% of water), but also an essential constituent of the organism, since water participates in many vital bodily functions, such as organ hydration, oxygen and nutrient transport in cells, toxin and waste elimination by the liver and kidneys, etc. Water also contributes to maintaining other important functions of the human body, such as the regulation of the body temperature and the lubrification of joints. In fact, water is so essential to the body that each of the cells that constitute it (including blood, lung, muscle, cartilage, skin, brain cells, and even bone cells) needs water to be able to live and function.

Since the body continuously eliminates water through the skin, respiration, perspiration and urine, the water lost by the body must be replaced by drinking enough water each day to provide enough water for each type of cells. When the ideal amount of water is reached, the cells are in a balanced and healthy environment and can therefore fully function. By contrast, as soon as the body lacks water (if only a little without provoking a feeling of thirst), this could cause a stress at the cell level. The most vulnerable body's cells will be affected first by a water deficiency and this will vary for each individual. Indeed, each of us has a weak point in terms of organ health. In one, it will be the cardiovascular system and the heart cells will be affected. In another, it will be the nervous system and the brain cells will be damaged. In yet another, it will be the respiratory system and the bronchi or the lungs will be affected. Or, it will be the skin and the dermis or epidermis will be weakened.

If the lack of water becomes chronic (that is, if it persists for several weeks or several months, or even for several years), the stress at the cell level could eventually spread to the different inter-cellular constituents and cause, depending on people, more or less serious diseases (like the ones described later in this chapter), affecting one of the organs mentioned above or another part of the body. Indeed, cells continually need enough water to maintain a healthy and favorable environment for the biochemical activities essential to life, whose activities are essentially fulfilled by proteins located mainly in, but also outside of cells. Proteins are key elements in the organism, where they fulfill varied and important functions. They play for example a crucial role in the maintenance of the cell structure, in the division of cells (e.g., for tissue regeneration), in the digestion of food, in the movement of muscles, in the immune defense, in respiration, in vision, etc. And, like cells, proteins need water to be able to fulfill their different functions and maintain the body in working condition.

I am a biochemist by training and have expertise in protein chemistry. My research studies, in several research laboratories of Swiss, French and American universities, as well as in laboratories of pharmaceutical and biotech companies, were conducted on numerous proteins, notably those involved in inflammatory diseases. The study of proteins is very useful for understanding diseases and for the development of medicines, but it can prove extremely complex. This is why, in order to simplify and facilitate their study, proteins are generally analyzed *in vitro*, which means outside the living organism or the cell. These analyses are carried out in vials or microtitration plates containing aqueous solutions that reproduce the physiological conditions inside the body. It turns out that if the amount of water in the vial is insufficient, the proteins will degrade and can form aggregates (sometimes visible by the naked eye) or precipitate suddenly, which prevents them from functioning normally.

A similar phenomenon may happen for proteins *in vivo*, i.e., inside the human body. Thus, when the amount of water in the body is insufficient, this may cause degradation and aggregation of proteins inside or outside of the cells. An important degradation of body's proteins for a prolonged period may be harmful and may cause illnesses in some persons due to protein dysfunction, such as Alzheimer's disease (abnormal aggregates of Tau protein in the brain), Parkinson's disease (accumulation of alpha-synuclein protein in the brain), osteoporosis (degradation of collagen proteins in bones), cataract (denaturation and agglutination of crystalline lens proteins in the eye), etc. By contrast, when proteins are in an environment that contains enough water to hydrate them, they can optimally fulfill their functions without degrading or aggregating, which may minimize or even prevent the onset of the diseases described above.

Water not only enables the hydration of the cells and the proteins that constitute the human body, but it also contributes to maintaining a balanced concentration of diverse molecules (such as carbohydrates, i.e., sugars; lipids, i.e., fat; hormones; etc.) that are present in the organism. A dehydrated body, which does not contain enough water, will thus have a higher concentration of molecules in blood or in cells than a well hydrated organism. To illustrate this point, let's take as an example a coffee prepared with two spoons of instant coffee and one spoon of sugar: the more the coffee is diluted with water, the lower the concentration of coffee and sugar, and vice-versa, the less the coffee contains water, the stronger the coffee with a high concentration of sugar and coffee.

So, by analogy, the concentration for example of the hormone cortisol will be higher in a dehydrated body, which lacks water. Cortisol (commonly called stress hormone) is a molecule that exerts diverse beneficial effects on the organism. This hormone stimulates inter alia the synthesis of glucose and regulates fat metabolism. However, too much cortisol in the blood (resulting for example from a dehydration of the organism, which will therefore induce a higher concentration of cortisol in the body) may be prejudicial to health and may cause in certain people a state of chronic stress, if this high level persists. Furthermore, too much stress hormone due to a dehydration of the body over a more or less long period may also increase anxiety in people who suffer from anxiety disorder or excessive worry. By contrast, a good body hydration will decrease the level of cortisol, which may consequently contribute to diminishing stress and calming anxiety states in people with these disorders (this could also prevent the development of other physical or mental health problems, such as bone mass loss or memory problems).

Cortisol is evidently not the only element of the body whose level increases when the amount of water in the organism diminishes. Several other molecules will also have a higher concentration in a dehydrated body, including for example toxins. A toxin is by definition a toxic substance for the organism. Thereby, too high a level of toxin, resulting here from a lack of water in the body, will produce harmful effects on the organism. These toxins being too concentrated could accumulate everywhere in the organism and cause in certain individuals health problems, such as for example chronic fatigue, migraines, insomnia, or even eczema (generally a minor yet embarrassing problem) if the toxins accumulate both in and on the skin. By contrast, an elevated level of toxins, or other molecules harmful to the body, will decrease in a well hydrated organism, since these molecules will be diluted by the water contained in the body, which will reduce their harmfulness.

In addition to maintaining a balanced and healthy level of components in the blood and in the cells of the human body, water also participates in the maintenance of a high performance immune system. Indeed, the immune system, which is a defense system of the organism against infections due to pathogenic elements (e.g., SARS-CoV-2, acronym for "Severe Acute Respiratory Syndrome Coronavirus 2", pneumococcal or tuberculosis bacteria, malaria parasite, etc.) or against foreign substances in the body, functions better with a sufficient intake of water, and a state of dehydration may weaken it. The body indeed needs enough fluid so as to be able to optimally humidify nasal and respiratory mucous membranes, and thereby rapidly and effectively clear away micro-organisms that attack it non-stop through respiratory tracts. Well hydrated and therefore well humidified mucous membranes have the ability to clear away viruses and other bacteria much more easily, thus avoiding colds, sore throats and other seasonal flus.

One of the reasons (among others) people get sick is the under-hydration of the organism. Indeed, if the body lacks some water (even just a little depending on the individuals), the nasal mucous membranes can get dehydrated or even dry (particularly in winter in buildings equipped with central heating, which dries the air), thereby decreasing the organism's ability to eliminate microbes that infect it. What's more, a dehydrated body is a weakened body and is therefore less able to destroy microbes, which have managed to pass the respiratory mucous membranes barrier, or which have penetrated through the digestive tract. This will prevent the organism from fighting efficiently against the infection and will allow microbes to multiply in the body and cause diseases.

In addition to all the diseases already mentioned in this chapter, other ailments and pathologies may also develop in certain people, due to a chronic lack of water in the body.

Here is a non-exhaustive list:
Acne
Bursitis (described in the first chapter)
Depression
Digestive problems (constipation, diarrheas, ulcers, etc.)
Gallstones
Gout
Hair loss
High and low blood pressure
Hypercholesterolemia (high cholesterol)
Menopause symptoms
Menstrual cramps (painful periods)
Plantar fasciitis (described in the first chapter)
Prostate problems
Tendinitis
Urinary tract infections
Uterine fibroids
Vasovagal syncope
Yeast infections.

Some diseases indicated in this list (e.g., bursitis, gout, tendinitis) are due to an inflammatory process. Other more serious, even potentially deadly, inflammatory diseases could also occur if the amount of water in the organism is frequently, or even always, insufficient. A constantly under-hydrated body could indeed eventually cause a chronic inflammatory condition that may trigger certain chronic inflammatory pathologies, such as rheumatoid arthritis, diabetes, multiple sclerosis, cancer, cardiovascular diseases, etc.

Therefore, in order to help prevent the outbreak of diseases and of other illnesses mentioned in this chapter or minimize their development, it is recommended to maintain a state of optimal hydration of the body by following the new hydration method presented in this book.

4 The medical benefits of the water-based health method

The medical benefits of this new health method are multiple. First, this innovative hydration method simply yet effectively helps protect against an invisible chronic bodily and potentially harmful dehydration (that could go completely unnoticed). Nowadays, this new water-based health method actually proves particularly important, since it can contribute to facilitating the management of sanitary crises by fighting for example the infectious Coronavirus Disease 2019 or COVID-19 caused by the SARS-CoV-2 virus. Indeed, this new method, which allows an optimal hydration of the organism at all times, strengthens the body and reinforces the immune system as described above in chapter 3. Not only well hydrated people are less susceptible to be infected by COVID-19, but they are less likely to die in case of coronavirus infection. The worldwide application of this health method could thereby limit SARS-CoV-2 infections and decrease the mortality due to COVID-19, as well as those associated with future potentially deadly infectious diseases.

In addition to optimizing the immune system and therefore fighting against infectious diseases, this new water-based health method can also relieve numerous relatively common illnesses, such as digestive disorders mentioned in the previous chapters (e.g., constipation, diarrhea, heartburn, etc.) or dermatologic disorders (e.g., rashes, psoriasis, hives, etc.). This new method may also prevent or alleviate eye floaters in the vitreous, also called floaters (which consists of aggregates of proteins or cell debris), as well as dry eye syndrome, since it keeps the organism fully hydrated, including the eyes.

This new health method may also alleviate asthma attacks and respiratory allergies by preventing bronchial tubes to dry up and by keeping them optimally hydrated at all times. This hydration method can also help prevent kidney stone formation, urinary tract infections, tendinitis or vasovagal syncope, since all these ailments result mainly from a dehydration of the organism. This water-based health method can also prevent strokes and heart attacks, since it optimizes the blood volume, which liquefies blood and facilitates its transport (accompanied by oxygen) to the organs.

Moreover, cancers could be avoided by applying this new health method, which helps minimize inflammatory conditions (notably due to chronic inflammation) often associated with cancers (clinical studies have actually shown an association between a limited consumption of water and the development of colorectal and breast cancers).

Furthermore, this water-based health method can prevent or alleviate depression in people prone to mood disorders, most particularly if the depressed person cries, because tears dehydrate the body, which exacerbates depression, i.e., the more we cry, the more we are dehydrated and the more we are depressed.

Patients suffering from Post-Traumatic Stress Disorder (PTSD) or from bipolar disorder could also benefit from this method, which helps regulate chemical substances of the brain and thus electrical signals and electrochemical reactions in neurons forming thoughts (particularly since the brain is composed of 80% water and is very vulnerable to dehydration). A water-based emergency treatment could actually be provided to patients in a state of psychiatric crisis (e.g., anxiety attack, psychosis, suicide attempt, etc.). The patient in a mental health crisis should therefore in the first place (if able of course) take one or several sips of water. This will allow a good hydration of the brain, which is very sensitive to water deficit, and thus help the sick person take the first step towards the stabilization of the mental health status and the consolidation of the post-crisis clinical remission. Moreover, this method can also fight against or even prevent sleep disorders (such as insomnia or nighttime awakenings) and/or alleviate persistent tiredness (permanent chronic fatigue causing a general feeling of exhaustion, which does not disappear with sleep or rest). This hydration method could even help people with addictive behaviors, such as alcoholism or drug addiction, since it creates some balance (or even a full balance) in the body and gives both mental and physical strength.

Another benefit of this new water-based health method is to relieve and prevent nocturnal leg cramps or exercise-associated cramps. Muscle cramps can be triggered for example during intense muscular exercise (notably with an accumulation of lactic acid in the muscles) or also during sleep at night while the body dehydrates naturally through the skin, breathing and sweating. The water supplied by this health method not only serves to eliminate the lactic acid in muscles, but also keeps the body hydrated overnight and therefore helps prevent cramps (which can sometimes be extremely painful). It should be noted that tennis players (who hydrate frequently during their match breaks) suffer very rarely from cramps, whereas soccer players (who play non-stop during 45 minutes or more) often have cramps particularly in summer when it is hot outside (and when the body eliminates a large amount of water through sweating).

This new water-based health method is also beneficial during airplane travels, where passengers dehydrate rapidly, since the airplane cabin air is very dry. The application of this health method before, during and after airplane travels, optimally hydrates the organism and liquefies blood, and may therefore prevent phlebitis, thrombosis or syncope resulting from air dryness in airplane cabins.

Moreover, this water-based health method is useful during medication intake or vaccine injection (for example COVID-19 vaccines). Indeed, the optimal hydration of the body and of all its organs optimizes the absorption and the distribution of the medicine or the vaccine (i.e., transport in blood and diffusion in tissues) and may thus help avoid (or at least minimize) adverse and undesirable effects, which may result from a water deficit in both cells and tissues, affecting the mechanism of action and the metabolism of drugs and vaccines. Therefore, if an allergic reaction occurs after the absorption of a medicine or the administration of a vaccine, even after several weeks or several months, the allergic symptoms (e.g., swelling and/or itching of the skin or of the mucous membranes, stuffy nose, respiratory problems, etc.) will be alleviated thanks to the beneficial effect of water and the optimal hydration of the body, and the symptoms will disappear more rapidly. This water-based health method is all the more beneficial during medication intake, when the drug's side effect is dehydration itself, since the goal of this method is to hydrate the body. This new method can thus counteract the harmful side effect of dehydration of these medicines.

Actually, this new water-based health method aims at reducing (or even stopping) medication intake, since it preserves an optimal hydration level of the body at all times and thus favors well-being and good health. A healthy body does not need medicines. It is however sometimes essential to take medicine (or get vaccinated, for example against COVID-19) and it is advisable, in that case, to apply the water-based health method described in this book, so as to optimize the action of the drug or vaccine in the body, and their elimination through the urine.

This new health method is particularly beneficial for the elderly. Indeed, the older we get, the more affected we are by poor body hydration, since the body contains, as it ages, less and less water with regard to the body mass (indeed, the elderly only have 45 to 50% water in their body, whereas a baby has 75% water, a child about 70%, and an adult 55-65% - a woman's body is composed in average of 50 to 55% water, while that of a man contains about 60 to 65%). Moreover, the older we get, the less we feel thirsty even if the body is dehydrated. The elderly are thereby more vulnerable to dehydration than a younger person and can often be in a state of chronic lack of water without even noticing it. The organism of an old person may therefore easily be dehydrated and susceptible to developing diseases. It is not necessarily aging that causes diseases and cancers, but rather dehydration of the organism. The regular consumption of small sips of water may therefore help the elderly to relieve rheumatisms, to avoid memory loss (e.g., Alzheimer's disease), to prevent cancer, to treat urinary incontinence, etc., and this without necessarily causing a more frequent need to urinate. I had an octogenarian friend, who practically did not drink anything, because she was in an electrical wheelchair and it was quite complicated for her to go to the toilet. She told me one day "if I drink, I have to often go to the bathroom and it is difficult with my wheelchair". Actually, this new water-based health method, with its regular and frequent sips of water, helps equilibrate the body and in particular the kidneys, and thus reduces the frequency of the need to urinate.

Another benefit (not necessarily medical but rather aesthetic) of this new method of hydration is the improvement of the skin and in particular the face (which is the part of the skin which dries out the more rapidly, since it is the most exposed to the environment, i.e., to the sun, the wind, the ambient dryness, for example due to heating systems in winter). Optimal hydration of the skin, thanks to this new method, can help avoid and alleviate skin problems, such as dry and oily skin, pimples of the face (for example whiteheads or pustules, or blackheads), rosacea, etc. This water-based health method can also reduce wrinkles, and prevent or reduce acne on the face (or on the back), as well as dark circles or bags under the eyes. This new method may also prevent or even diminish cellulitis on the thighs or the stretch marks on the belly, the hips and the breasts.

Although this new water-based health method can help manage diseases and symptoms associated with various health problems, disease prevention is of course simpler to realize and easier to apply than healing, even with this innovative health method. Indeed, the old proverb "prevention is better than cure" is still quite relevant today. It is therefore preferable to apply this hydration method before the appearance of the first signs or symptoms of a disease or an ailment, but one must certainly not give up if the disease is already present, because this new health method can lessen the harm and stabilize or even heal diseases depending on their level of severity.

This new water-based health method is highly beneficial for the human body, since it is actually not easy to know if our organism – and thus our cells, our organs and our blood – lack water and suffer from dehydration. It is indeed quite difficult to measure the degree of bodily dehydration. With the exception of a dark yellow colored urine (when the body is already deeply dehydrated), along with sometimes (but not always) a dry mouth and a feeling of thirst, it is practically impossible to determine if we are dehydrated or not (there aren't currently rapid, inexpensive and accurate tests to detect body dehydration, particularly if it is mild or moderate). The sensation of thirst is supposed to alert the organism of the lack of water in order to incite it to renew its water reserves, but this sensation does not always manifest itself. This lack of feeling of thirst may be due to a lack of physical activity associated with our modern way of life. Indeed nowadays, most of us work sitting at a desk often with air-conditioning and stay at the same place for hours without any physical activity. After our workday, we go home by car or by public transportation and do little or no physical exercise. This lack of physical activity can compromise our sensation of thirst and thus generate a state of dehydration without even knowing it. In the past, thanks to physical labor (for example in the fields, to wash clothes, etc.), we probably felt thirst more (indeed, just doing housework or going for a walk – particularly in summer – can make you thirsty), but now with the appearance of electrical appliances for domestic use (e.g., washing machines or dishwashers, vacuums, lawn mowers, etc.) and with the urbanization due to the development of society towards industry and services, our sedentary lifestyles make us feel less thirsty.

As it is not obvious to know if our body is dehydrated or not, the implementation of the new water-based health method, described in chapter 2, helps keep an optimal hydration of the organism at all times and may thus improve the general state of health in order to be (and remain) in good health.

5 The financial benefits of the water-based health method

Considering that this new water-based health method, which helps keep an optimal hydration of the organism at all time, may improve the general health status, the number of sick people in the world could decrease. Thanks to this new health method, people would go less to the doctor or to the hospital and they would consume less medication, since they would be in better shape. The number of ill people would therefore decrease and the number of healthy people would increase, which would *de facto* contribute to reducing healthcare costs.

Healthcare spending is handled by public services (e.g., Medicare and Medicaid in the U.S.), by private health insurances (and in certain countries also by employers), but also by the individuals themselves by direct payment for their own care. The expenses are significant for public services and for the individuals, and may reach hundreds of thousands of dollars per person for the span of a lifetime or even for a single specific treatment, in particular for the biological medicines or the new cell and gene therapies with individualized care.

Healthcare costs are mainly due to chronic diseases (e.g., arthritis, diabetes, cancers, etc.), which are quite often avoidable and may generally be avoided with a healthy lifestyle (i.e., regular physical activity without tobacco or excess alcohol) and with a healthy diet (i.e., balanced meals composed of fruits and vegetables without any excess of sugar, salt or fat). A healthy diet also includes an adequate consumption of water, so as to optimally hydrate the body. If the public authorities (including hospitals) incite and help people drink more water thanks to this new health method, this would allow them to usefully and advantageously manage the evolution of healthcare costs (particularly in order to regulate the prices imposed by medical services and pharmaceutical groups). Moreover, if this simple and effective health method is applied worldwide, this could help all the countries reduce healthcare spending globally (since it seems that nowadays the global standardization of sanitary conditions contributes to increasing healthcare spending). We would furthermore use less (or in a more targeted way) costly technical medical innovations, which would also contribute to decreasing healthcare spending.

A reduction in healthcare expenditure would prove most beneficial to society, since global healthcare costs are constantly increasing every year, mainly because of ageing population, which is accompanied by an increase of pathologies and therefore costs. It should be noted that healthcare spending during the pandemic of

COVID-19 has greatly increased. Thanks to this new water-based health method, people would actually be in better health and would stay healthy longer and longer. The socioeconomic repercussions would be considerable with major financial benefits (i.e., lower Medicare/Medicaid costs, reduction of medical fees, health insurance premium and co-pay relief, etc.). This would be beneficial for everyone: healthy people in good shape, as well as less fit people.

6 The choice of water

The health method described in this book is based on water and more particularly on the frequent consumption of sips of water in order to maintain the body hydrated at all times. But, which water is appropriate to drink all day long? There are indeed several types of water, such as tap water, mineral water (from an underground origin and of stable chemical composition that may have therapeutic effects), spring water (from an underground origin without chemical treatment), sparkling water (with addition of carbon dioxide gas), plain water (mineral or spring water that does not contain gas), etc. All these types of water can be bottled and sold commercially (including tap water, which is filtered before being bottled). The bottles of water are generally in plastic (sometimes 100% recycled and often recyclable) or in glass (in the past returnable and progressively replaced by plastic), and since a few years ago, bottles in paperboard or in metal (i.e., aluminum) are also available in certain stores.

There are advantages and disadvantages for each type of water. The main advantage of tap water is its easy consumption at home or at work, since it is available 24/7, simply by turning on the kitchen faucet (except of course in case of water service interruptions, which fortunately rarely occur). Another not negligible advantage is its low price, therefore accessible to all. Moreover tap water, which is treated and highly controlled in developed countries, has in general a low level of minerals and therefore does not overload the body with chemical elements potentially harmful to certain people. The major disadvantage of tap water is its taste due to chlorine, which is added to disinfect water and to limit growth of microorganisms (such as bacteria or viruses).

The chlorine taste may however dissipate by letting the water run for a few minutes, before filling a pitcher that should be kept in the fridge during a minimum of 30 minutes so that water can aerate. Before drinking tap water, it is necessary to always let the water run for a few minutes until it is cold, so as to avoid drinking water that has stagnated in pipes (and that could be contaminated with materials from pipes).

If pollutants in tap water are a concern (such as lead coming from old pipes in older houses), water may be filtered and purified with a water filter pitcher commercially available. In order to maintain an acceptable quality of water in the filter pitcher, it has to be frequently cleaned and the filter must be changed often (by following the instructions from the vendor). Moreover, the pitcher should be kept in the refrigerator and the water should be consumed within 24 hours, so as to avoid in particular the growth of microorganisms in the pitcher (since chlorine is not only filtered, but also eliminated by aeration). Although tap water is subject to very strict quality criteria before being distributed to the consumers, there are sometimes exceptional cases of contaminated water (for example by bacteria or by chemical products). It is then necessary to get bottles of water until the tap water contamination is totally eliminated. In case of contamination only by microorganisms, the tap water may be boiled before being consumed (in this case, water must be boiled to a rolling boil during at least 1 minute, so as to kill all the germs).

Contrary to tap water, which is subject to disinfection treatments, so as to become drinkable (notably by addition of chlorine), mineral water as well as spring water (which have their underground origin free of any pollution) are not disinfected. Indeed, mineral waters and spring waters meet specific requirements and are naturally not polluted. Another advantage of mineral waters is their low or high mineralized composition, since mineral water, as the name suggests, may contain a lot of minerals (for example water with high sulfate, bicarbonate or magnesium levels, or by contrast low in salt). Thereby, certain mineral waters, by their specific and stable composition, are characterized by therapeutic qualities. However, it should be pointed out that mineral waters with a high level of minerals may be contraindicated for example in case of high blood pressure, heart failure or kidney failure. Moreover, sparkling mineral waters can irritate the colon and cause bloating or flatulence (intestinal gas).

Since mineral and spring waters are generally bottled, their main disadvantage is the ecological and environmental impact due to bottle waste, especially those in non-recyclable plastic, since plastic is particularly harmful to the environment. Plastic bottles may not only pollute the planet, but they may also endanger health, since water contained in certain plastic bottles is contaminated by tiny plastic particles (micro- and nano-plastic originating from the bottles themselves), which could be harmful. The environmental impact of water bottles is also due to their transport (from bottling to recycling), causing non-negligible emissions of CO_2 (carbon dioxide), one of the main greenhouse gases. Moreover, contrary to tap water which is available directly in a glass or in a pitcher in unlimited amount, water bottles are relatively heavy to carry from the grocery store (or from the car) to the house particularly for the elderly. Both mineral and spring waters also have a downside in terms of cost, since their price is much higher than that of tap water. If bottled water is preferred, it is important to ensure a sufficient supply of bottles is available at home. Likewise, if tap water is preferred, it is also advisable to keep at least 1 gallon of bottled water at home per person, so as to always have water to drink even during water service interruptions.

So, among all these types of water, should we favor one in particular? There aren't really any rules. Tap water and bottled water may for example be alternatively consumed by drinking for instance tap water at home and bottled mineral or spring water at work or when going to a restaurant, the movies or a concert. The important thing is simply to drink water by applying the health method described in this book. It is however necessary to take into account the high levels of minerals and salts of certain mineral waters, which are not suitable for people suffering for example (as mentioned above) from high blood pressure or kidney failure. Moreover, if flatulence is a concern, still water can be favored over sparkling water. However, if sparkling water is preferred, it can be consumed all day long (except in case of contraindications to carbonated water), the most important thing is to regularly take a sip of water (even sparkling water) approximately every 30 minutes, rather than not drinking at all on the pretext that we do not like still water. There are also nowadays in stores many flavored sparkling waters (with natural fruit flavors) without sugar or sweetener, which may be consumed as part of this new water-based health method. Since the goal of this health method consist of taking sips of water all day long, it is necessary to choose a water that we enjoy drinking. Drinking water is a privilege in developed market-economy countries, so let's enjoy it!

7 Conclusion

As explained in the previous chapters, many diseases and ailments result mainly from a chronical and recurrent dehydration of the organism. The human body must indeed be continuously in an optimal aqueous environment, otherwise it may stop functioning optimally. In a constantly dehydrated (even slightly under-hydrated) organism, all the cells, which compose it, are dehydrated to a greater or lesser degree according to the type of cells (those from the lungs, the brain, the skin, etc.) and are thereby in an almost permanent state of stress and tension depending on the level of dehydration of the body, which could cause a dysfunction of the cells at the level of their proteins (as described above), of their DNA (i.e., chromosomes), of their membranes, etc. The constant lack of water prevents cells from fulfilling their normal functions of body maintenance. This cell dysregulation (resulting from the lack of water in the body) may spread to organs formed by cells and lead to their degradation and deterioration with dire consequences on health.

By contrast, numerous diseases and illnesses may be prevented by always keeping our body well hydrated in an optimal state of water balance, so as to continuously enable the well-being of all the cells composing the organism and thereby the proper functioning of organs. Indeed, diseases have the potential to be prevented, stabilized or cured with a sufficient intake of water in the organism, whether it is a viral infection (such as the common cold or the more deadly COVID-19), diabetes, depression, high blood pressure or a potentially more serious illness, such as heart failure or cancer. By regularly drinking water and thus keeping the body hydrated throughout the day (and therefore throughout the night, thanks to the beneficial hydration of the day), people could prevent or even cure diseases. In particular, thanks to this new water-based health method described in the chapter 2 of this booklet (and to its frequent and regular sips of water), it is possible to benefit from an optimal hydration of the body and of all its organs at any moment of the day and of the night, and thereby alleviate or even eliminate health or mental problems (or even prevent their appearance) and accelerate healing.

Yet, I have noticed that a lot of people rarely drink between meals except perhaps a coffee in the morning around 10 a.m. or some tea in the afternoon around 4 p.m., for example during work breaks (which actually tends to dehydrate the organism). Many people therefore stay for hours without fluid intake to replace the loss of water (which has been stored - as urine - in the bladder, or evaporated in ambient air through the skin, sweat and breathing, especially during the summer when it is hot). They thereby unintentionally dry out their body and thus all the cells that compose it. With the influx of fluid from food and beverages at noon and in the evening, their body is hydrated for a certain time, and then finds itself in a state of chronic dehydration (especially if the amount of fluid consumed during meals is insufficient).

Unfortunately, the majority of people nowadays do not take time to drink water and above all they do not think of hydrating themselves, or they do not wish to drink too much water due to worries about having to go to the bathroom all the time. Therefore, they sometimes stay for hours without drinking water and are thus in a state of under-hydration, which can potentially be deleterious for health. For example, I have recently read on social media that an athlete suggested to another athlete, who apparently suffered from cramps, to drink water (she did not even know, she did not think of it, she thanked her). Moreover, during a recent outdoor music concert in the summer, I noticed that no one was hydrating around me although the outside temperature was close to 86°F. Furthermore, I sometimes hear friends or acquaintances say that they went to the emergency room because they fainted. Yet, the diagnosis is often acute dehydration with, as emergency care an intravenous fluid perfusion. I myself did not hydrate sufficiently several years ago and I suffered from frequent digestion problems (fortunately without having to go to the hospital). I also frequently caught colds. This would start with a sore throat, which would turn into a cold and inevitably end with a stubborn cough. One day I had the idea to frequently take little sips of water. Actually, ever since I drink water according to my method described in this book, I have not suffered from digestive disorders and rarely fall ill, and if I nevertheless catch a cold, symptoms are light and do not last and I am not afflicted with a persistent cough during several weeks.

Everyone can actually benefit from this new water-based health method, which (associated with a healthy lifestyle, including a minimum of physical activity and a good eating habit) keeps you in shape and healthy throughout life. Moreover, this new health method is natural and easy to apply. Furthermore, it does not make you fat and may even contribute to losing weight during weight loss diets and to facilitating stabilization of one's ideal weight after a slimming diet. It is however necessary, in certain cases, to discuss this hydration method with a primary care doctor, so as to ensure that there aren't any medical restrictions limiting the application of this new water-based health method.

It should be noted that this new health method may probably not prevent and heal all the diseases, but it may certainly contribute to alleviating ailments and reducing various medical problems potentially deadly, and even prevent death caused by certain illnesses. It is indeed not guaranteed that this water-based health method is suitable and successful for everyone, this will depend on the gravity of the disease. That being said, there isn't really any disadvantage to follow this hydration method, but there are on the other hand many advantages to put it into practice. In fact, to fully benefit from the advantages of this water-based health method, it is advisable to (as mentioned above) maintain a healthy lifestyle (by practicing a physical activity) and eat a healthy and balanced diet (by favoring fruits and vegetables, with enough vitamins and minerals, and without too much sugar, saturated fat and salt).

Finally yet importantly, this innovative health method could contribute to preventing future pandemics and save lives, since people being optimally hydrated, would be in better shape and healthier. Especially since this water-based health method is very easy to follow at home, since we can easily drink tap water or even bottles of water delivered directly at home.

This health method is for everyone: for both women and men, and for young and old alike, but it is particularly aimed at the elderly, who no longer feel thirst and who are worried about having to go to the bathroom too often. Everyone indeed wishes to live in great shape and in good health. The old saying goes "As long as you've got your health!". Yet, this method can help each and every one prevent diseases or even cure some. So, let's hydrate!

Afterword

Hydration is crucial for health. Yet, half of the world's population does not drink the recommended amounts of fluid and a large majority of Americans are chronically dehydrated.

Dehydration is quite often overlooked and inadequately prevented, particularly since its assessment can be a challenge due to a complex physiology, non-specific clinical presentation, and limitations on diagnostic methods and testing.

The new water-based health method presented by Dr. Sibyl Baladi can help prevent dehydration and also optimize body hydration. In addition to helping people improve body hydration thanks to her innovative yet simple method, Dr. Baladi has another mission: to develop a new and affordable rapid test that will accurately determine hydration status (with a novel objective marker of dehydration).

Altogether, this should contribute to optimizing the assessment, management, prevention and treatment of dehydration, and thus improving health and wellness.